I0449857

The History of Dietetics

John B. Nichols
Felix L. Oswald

The History of Dietetics

Man is what he eats

LM Publishers

The history of dietetics[1]

The manifold diversities in diet, the articles employed as food, the manner of preparing food, customs of eating, etc…, among different peoples and at different times have been the outcome of fortuitous evolution, unguided and uninfluenced by definite physiologic principles. An account of the development of such dietary practises would present much of interest and would be included in a complete history of dietetics; but it is far too large a subject to be considered here, and the present paper will be limited to a brief presentation of the development of the various lines of knowledge constituting the scientific basis of dietetics, as it exists today.

Inquiring and speculative minds in all ages have endeavored to trace out the principles and laws governing diet. Prior to the modern scientific era, that is, during the entire ancient and middle ages, there was very little foundation of real knowledge on which a true science of dietetics could be based. Only the crudest objective characteristics of foodstuffs could be appreciated, such as the

---

[1] By John B. Nichols

7

division of animal and vegetable, liquid and solid, etc. Notwithstanding the want of any adequate basis, from the time of Hippocrates a large proportion of medical literature was devoted to the subject of dietetics, and a multitude of treatises on food were presented characterized by chimerical speculation and fine-spun theorizing. Mythical properties and dangers were ascribed to different foodstuffs; rules were laid down in minute detail as to the use or prohibition of various foods in different morbid conditions which were without rational warrant; dietetic theories and systems were propounded which in the light of modern knowledge are seen to have been grotesque; and the authorities expounded their doctrines with an emphasis and dogmatism paralleled only by their real ignorance of the subject. Of all the mass of dietetic doctrine presented in the ancient and medieval eras of medical thought, there was very little of abiding verity or value that contributed to our present rational knowledge of the subject. On the contrary, the professional mind was thoroughly indoctrinated with erroneous ideas which retarded the acceptance of correct conceptions and have not even yet been eradicated.

The science of dietetics is a composite subject, uniting a number of rather independent branches of knowledge, such as the chemistry of food, the processes of digestion, the physiology of metabolism, etc., the development of which may be separately considered. The beginnings of our scientific knowledge of these subjects may be traced back to the seventeenth century, soon after the discovery of the circulation of the blood by William Harvey (1578-1667), announced in 1628, opened the way to the development of scientific physiology. Xo great progress, however, was made for nearly two centuries, and the main foundations of our knowledge of these subjects were laid down in the second quarter of the nineteenth century.

The development of our knowledge of the physiology of digestion will be first considered.

A knowledge of the mechanism of glandular secretion in general is prerequisite to an understanding of the origin of the digestive fluids. No adequate conception of the structure and function of glands was possible prior to the discovery of the circulation and the use of the microscope. "When these conditions were fulfilled the physiology' of glandular secretion was quickly worked out. At first, for instance, it was not even known that, except for the liver and kidneys, the glands possessed ducts. The main steps in the evolution of our knowledge of glandular action were about as follows :

In 1643 the duct of the pancreas was first described by Georg Wirsung, a Bavarian (died 1643), although his pupil Maurice Hoffmann contested the honor of its discovery as his own. In 1654 Francis Glisson, an Englishman (1597-1677), published an important work on the liver, in which he touched upon the mechanism of the secretion of the bile. In 1656 Thomas Wharton, an Englishman (1610-1673), published an account of the duct of the submaxillary gland. In 1662 Lorenzo Bellini, of Florence (1643-1704), at the early age of 19 years, described certain portions of the uriniferous tubules of the kidney. In 1663 also Nicolas Stensen, or Steno, a Dane (1638-1686), described the ducts of the parotid and other glands. The names of these observers have ever since been attached to the structures which they discovered.

About this time Franciscus Sylvius, Stenscn's instructor at Leyden, drew a general distinction between conglomerate glands, possessing secretory ducts, such as ordinary secreting glands, and conglobate glands, such as the lymphatic glands. Stensen, from his researches on the salivary and other glands, came close to an adequate conception of the process of glandular secretion ; but as, like the other observers just mentioned, he did not employ the microscope, he was unable to work out the full details of the subject. It remained for

Marcello Malpighi (1628-1694), of Bologna, a pioneer microscopist and one of the first and greatest of histologists, in 1666 to lay down finally the essential features of the minute structure and mechanism of the main glandular organs as they are accepted at the present time.

The lacteals were discovered in 1622 (published 1627) by Gaspare Aselli (1581-1626), professor at Pavia, who recognized that they conveyed the chyle away from the intestine, but regarded them as emptying into the liver, then thought to be the organ in which the food materials were converted into blood. The discovery of the receptaculum chyli and the thoracic duct, and the connection of these with the lacteals on the one hand, and the venous system on the other, was made independently by Jean Pecquet (1622-1674), of Dieppe and Paris, and Jan van Home (1621-1670), of Leyden, whose observations were published in 1651 and 1652, respectively.

In the ancient and middle ages, the stomach was looked upon as the principal organ of digestion. The process of digestion was by some (Hippocrates and others) regarded as a coction, or 77^15 (cooking), a sort of maturation effected with the aid of heat; by others it was considered as akin to putrefaction; and by still others as a mechanical process. It came to be the general doctrine that the food material absorbed from the alimentary tract was first acted upon by the liver and endowed with "natural spirits" ; in the heart, by the action on the blood of the inspired air, the natural spirits were converted into "vital spirits"; finally, in the brain the vital spirits were converted into "animal spirits," which were then conveyed by the nerves to all parts of the body.

The beginnings of our modern knowledge of digestion can be traced back to the observations of the Belgian savant Jean Baptiste van Helmont (1577-1644), whose work formed a landmark in the history of chemistry. He regarded the chemical activities of the body as a form of fermentation, analogous to the familiar alcoholic or vinous fermentation; he assigned ferment action as a cause of a wide range of vital processes, thus anticipating theories that at the present time are frequently advanced. In van Helmont's view the digestion of food was accomplished by fermentative action. He recognized only two stages of digestion in the alimentary tract, namely, in the stomach and in the duodenum; the action of the salivary glands and pancreas was not yet known. Gastric digestion he regarded as being effected by a ferment derived from the spleen, associated with an acid principle which was necessary to its action. When the chyme passed into the duodenum the acid ferment was neutralized, and the second stage of digestion was effected by the bile.

The next developments in the knowledge of digestion came from Franciscus Sylvius (Frangois de la Boe, or Dubois, 1614-1672), the professor of medicine at Leyden, who founded the iatro-ehemical school and exerted a powerful influence as a teacher and expositor of the chemical philosophy of his time. Sylvius also attributed many of the vital processes to fermentative action; but he confused effervescence (such as occurs on adding acid to carbonate) with fermentation, and looked upon effervescence as the type of these processes. Sylvius had knowledge of two secretions, salivary and pancreatic, unknown to van Helmont.

The observations of Wharton and Stensen (published 1656 and 1662) had clarified the salivary secretion. Impressed with these discoveries, Sylvius attached an exaggerated importance to the digestive action of the saliva, and held that digestion in the stomach was accomplished much more by swallowed saliva than by any ferment of gastric origin. This view persisted for a long time.

The second stage of digestion, that taking place in the duodenum, according to Sylvius was effected by the conjoint action of the bile and the recently discovered pancreatic juice. Wirsung in 1643 had described the pancreatic duct; and in 1664 Regner de Graaf (1641-1673), of Holland, published the results of investigations on the pancreatic secretion carried out while he was a student at Leyden under Sylvius. De Graaf obtained pure pancreatic juice from dogs through quills inserted into the pancreatic duct. He fell into the error, however, of regarding it as acid; and he held, in accordance with Sylvius's theory of effervescence, that the effervescence supposed to be produced by the mixture of this acid juice with the salts of the bile was in some way associated with duodenal digestion.

In 1677, Johann Conrad Peyer (1653-1712), a Swiss, published a description of certain glandular structures discovered by him and since known as Peyer's patches. He decided that these were secretory (conglomerate) rather than lymphatic (conglobate) glands, and believed their secretion had digestive properties, active in the lower ileum at a point where the pancreatic juice must become exhausted.

In 1683, Johann Conrad Brunner (1653-1727), of Germany, published the results of experiments which he had made in exsecting the pancreas and ligating the pancreatic duct in dogs. As the dogs did not manifest any disturbance of digestion or nutrition, he argued that the importance attached by Sylvius and de Graaf to pancreatic digestion was unfounded. Brunner also showed that the pancreatic juice was not acid. In 1687 he described the duodenal glands, since known by his name, and attributed digestive properties to their secretion.

In consequence of the doubt brought by the discoveries of Peyer and Brunner, belief in pancreatic digestion waned, and for a long time the view prevailed that the stomach was the chief seat of digestion. In the latter part of the seventeenth century, two opposing theories as to the mechanism of gastric digestion were held by the rival physical and chemical schools of that period. The chemical theory of digestion was that of van Helmont, Sylvius, and their followers. On the other hand, Alfonso Borelli (1608-1679), the founder of the iatro-physical school, held that gastric secretion was chiefly effected by powerful trituration of the ingested food by the muscular walls of the stomach, as appears especially in birds; and while he conceded a corrosive action of the stomach juices in some species, his followers denied all chemical digestion and regarded the Avhole process as purely mechanical.

During the eighteenth century the only additions to the knowledge of digestion were a few studies of the gastric juice.

Rene Antoine Ferchault de Reaumur (1683-1757) developed a new and fruitful method of investigation, publishing his results in 1753. He introduced metal tubes containing various food materials into the stomach of a buzzard (which, like other carnivorous birds, ejects from the mouth indigestible substances like bones, etc.) and other animals, and on examining them subsequently was able to determine the effect of the gastric juice on these materials. By using sponges in the tubes he was the first to obtain gastric juice in pure condition. He observed that meat and bone were dissolved by the gastric juice, but not grains or flour. He thus demonstrated that this secretion possessed a definite solvent power, distinct from putrefaction, and independent of trituration.

Employing Reaumur's and other similar methods, Lazaro Spallanzani (1729-1799), of Italy, continued and extended the observations, publishing his results in 1777 and subsequently. In 1777 Stevens, of Edinburgh, published a similar research. John Hunter (1728-1793) in 1773 and 1786 also published some observations on digestion.

The acidity of the gastric juice, appreciated by van Helmont and denied by his successors, was not generally recognized until the nineteenth century. Spallanzani and Hunter regarded the acidity of some of the specimens which they obtained as occasional or exceptional or abnormal only. Carminati recognized the real conditions, showing in 1785 that the gastric juice while fasting is neutral, and is acid only after taking food; his observations, however, did not gain general attention,

A contribution of interest to Americans, which, however, passed unnoticed, was the graduation thesis of John R. Young, of Maryland, at the University of Pennsylvania in 1803, in which he described experiments made on digestion in the stomachs of frogs and human subjects, and demonstrated the acidity of the gastric juice.

The foundations of our present knowledge of digestion were mainly established during the second quarter of the nineteenth century.

William Prout (1785-1850), of London, in 1834 identified the acid principle of the gastric juice as hydrochloric acid.

William Beaumont (1785-1853), an American army surgeon, from 1825 to 1833 conducted a celebrated series of observations of gastric digestion through a fistula following a gunshot wound in the case of the Canadian Alexis Saint Martin, the results being published in 1833, These observations constituted an important contribution to the subject and attracted world-wide attention.

Leuchs in 1831 discovered the starch-digesting properties of saliva. Payen and Persoz in ISSS discovered and studied the amylolytic ferment diastase in germinating barley. Mialhe in 1845 isolated ptyalin from saliva.

J. N. Eberle in a work published in 1834 was the first to note the power of an extract or artificial gastric juice prepared from the gastric mucous membrane to dissolve proteid material. He, however, erroneously attributed this solvent action to the mucus on the surface of the stomach. Theodor Schwann (1810-1882), the discoverer of animal cells, investigated the subject (partly in association with his teacher Johannes Mliller) and in crude form isolated from the gastric mucosa a principle possessing intense proteolytic powers, to which he gave the name pepsin; his results were published in 1836.

In his treatise published in 1834 Eberle noted the fact that a watery extract of the pancreas would emulsify oil, and he surmised that one of the functions of the pancreatic secretion was to favor the absorption of fat. In 1836 Purkinje and Pappenheim discovered that extracts from the pancreas possess proteolytic properties. In 1844 Valentin made some observations on the starch-digesting powers of the pancreatic fluid; and in 1845 Bouchardat and Sandras definitely demonstrated the secretion of an amylolytic principle by this organ.

Following these pioneer discoveries, the elucidation of the functions of the pancreas, especially its fat-splitting action, was accomplished chiefly by the work of the French investigator Claude Bernard (1813- 1878), whose researches on this subject were prosecuted about 1836- 1846.

From these beginnings the chemistry and physiology of digestion have been further elaborated by numerous subsequent investigators.

The study of gastric digestion was made a simple clinical procedure by the employment of the stomach tube for obtaining samples of gastric juice. This originated with Adolph Kussmaul (18'22-190'2), who in 1869 reported the use of the stomach tube in the treatment of dilatation of the stomach; subsequent to which the examination of gastric juice for diagnostic purposes was elaborated by "W. 0. Leube, C. A. Ewald and Franz Riegel, and their associates during the seventies and eighties of the last century.

Important studies of the action of the digestive organs were not long ago made by Ivan Pyotrovich Pavlofl (often transliterated, from the German, J. P. Pawlow) (born 1849), director of the Imperial Institute of Experimental Medicine in Saint Petersburg, the results of whose brilliant researches (conducted

1887-1897) were first published in collected form in 1897. For this work Pavloff received the Nobel prize in 1904.

The discovery of pancreatic secretin by William Maddock Bayliss and Ernest Henry Starling, announced in 1904, opened up an entirely new field of knowledge, that of the action of the so-called hormones as inciters of secretory activity carried to the points of action by the circulation.

The introduction of the X-ray made available a new and fertile method of studying the movements of the digestive organs; one of the earliest and most prolific workers in this field has been an American, Walter Bradford Cannon, professor of physiology at Harvard, whose contributions on this subject date from 1899.

The main basis of dietetics rests in the chemistry of food and nutrition. This knowledge could not be developed until the science of chemistry entered upon its renaissance, which occurred much later than the birth of modern anatomy, physiology and physics. The discovery of oxygen in 1774 opened the way to a rapid development of chemical knowledge, just as Harvey's discovery of the circulation a century and a half before had been the starting point for physiology.

As has been the case with many other discoveries, the effective discovery of oxygen had been anticipated long previously by work that had fallen into oblivion. In 1668 a young Englishman at Oxford, John Mayow (1645-1679), published a remarkable work in which he argued that the atmosphere contains, as he styled it, an "igneo-aereal" or "nitro-aereal" principle which by combining with combustible ("sulphureous") substances constitutes the process of combustion; that this principle is imparted to the blood by the respiratory activities ; that the union of this principle, carried in the blood, with combustible material in the muscles gives rise to muscular action and is a source of animal heat. Though this theory was soon forgotten, it was a remark- able presentation of the doctrine of oxidation (including body oxidation as the source of animal energy), and anticipated by a century the discovery of oxygen.

In 1774 oxygen was independently discovered by Joseph Priestley (1733-1804), an English clergyman, and by Karl Wilhelm Scheele (1742-1786), of Sweden. It was Antoine Laurent Lavoisier (1743- 1794), of Paris, however, who grasped the real significance of this discovery, and by his researches, published from 1775, overthrew the false though fruitful phlogistic theory of heat that had dominated chemistry for a century, and showed the true nature of combustion and the properties of oxygen.

Lavoisier was followed by a number of brilliant investigators, who rapidly laid down the great foundations of chemical science. The beginnings of organic chemistry may be traced to some of these early workers; Lavoisier, for instance, showed that organic compounds are composed mainly of carbon, hydrogen and oxygen, and sometimes nitrogen.

The foundation and elaboration of organic chemistry was mainly the great achievement of the illustrious chemist Justus Liebig (1803-1873). After studying chemistry at Paris under Gay-Lussac, he was professor of chemistry at Giessen 1824-1852, and at Munich from 1853 until his death in 1873. About 1837 he began epoch-making investigations of physiologic and organic chemistry, and in works published from 1840 he laid down the main lines of our knowledge of the chemistry of food and nutrition. He first, for instance, sharply differentiated the foodstuffs albumen, fat and carbohydrate, and recognized the tissue- forming function of albumins and the heat-producing properties of fats and carbohydrates.

Since the time of Liebig many workers have brought our knowledge of the chemistry of food to its present state. Among important investigations of this character now being actively prosecuted are those on the molecular structure of the complex foodstuffs, such as the studies of Emil Fischer, Emil Abderhalden and others on the proteins. Some of the sugars have been artificially synthesized, and a beginning has been made even on the proteins.

Crude attempts at food analysis date back for centuries, as in connection with governmental measures to prevent adulteration of foods and beverages. In the modern era George Pearson, of England, in 1795 reported an analysis of potatoes; in 1805, Einhoff analyses of potatoes and rye. Reliable analyses of milk were reported by Peligot in 1836, and of feeding stuffs and milk by Boussingault and Le Bel 1836-1839. From about 1840, through the work of Liebig a great impetus was given to food analysis; and with the further advances of chemistry came the development of reliable analytic methods and the accumulation of data. From about 1860 the standard methods of food analysis now employed were developed by Wilhelm Henneberg (1825-1890), of the agricultural experiment station at Weende, near Gottingen; these methods soon came into general use and have greatly facilitated and S3'stematized this line of work.

Possibly the earliest analyses of food made in the United States were of some cereals by C. U. Shepherd published in 1844. Analyses of various foods were published by Salisbury in 1848, Beck in

1848-1849, Emmons in 1849, Jackson in 1857. One of the most prolific workers in this field in this country was Atwater, who, employing the Weende methods, made analyses of maize in 1869, and commenced an extended series of analyses of fish and other foods in 1877.

Dietary studies — investigations of the amounts of foodstuffs actually consumed by different classes of people under various conditions — furnish an important part of the data underlying the science of dietetics. Among the earliest investigations of this sort were those conducted by Liebig in 1810; by Beneke in England in 1851; and in this country by John Stanton Gould in 1852 and Atwater in 1886. Since then many such studies have been made and a large amount of information collected.

A knowledge of the processes of metabolism forms another component of the foundations of dietetics.

Probably the earliest real metabolism studies were prosecuted by Sanctorius (1561-1636), who published his results in 1614. Sitting in a chair suspended from steelyards, he observed the changes in weight from eating and from the loss of insensible perspiration.

Theories of the source of animal heat were presented from the early days of physiology. Van Helmont held that animal heat was generated by fermentation of the blood in the heart. Sylvius believed it to be produced by the supposed effervescence resulting from the mixture of venous blood with acid chyle. Mayow in 1668 anticipated the modern view that the body energy is derived from oxidation in the tissues; but his views were soon forgotten. Toward the end of the seventeenth century these chemical theories were largely superseded by the physical view that animal heat is generated by the friction of the blood in the capillaries. It was not until after the discovery of oxygen that our present conceptions of the part played by oxidation as the source of animal energy were founded by Lavoisier.

The general outlines of our knowledge of metabolism were formulated by Liebig, the details being worked out by numerous subsequent investigators, many of them under his personal influence. In this way, chiefly since 1850, an extensive mass of data on this subject has been accumulated. The earliest metabolism study appears to have been one by Lehmann, made in 1839. The study of the metabolism of nitrogen is a comparatively simple matter, and has been an easy and frequent subject for investigation.

The determination of the exchanges of carbon and hydrogen is a much more difficult matter, involving the collection of the products of respiration and requiring elaborate apparatus and an amount of labor rarely available. Early respiration experiments with animals were made by Boussingault about 1844, Bidder and Schmidt in 1847-1850, and Regnault and Reiset in 1849; and with man by Barral in 1847-1848, and Hildesheim in 1856.

A most extensive and accurate series of investigations was con- ducted by Max von Pettenkofer (1818-1901) and, especially, Carl von Yoit (1831-1908), in the Physiological Institute at Munich with the respiration apparatus constructed by Pettenkofer about 1860. Animals and men were made the subjects of extended observation with this apparatus from 1861 to 1867, and principles of fundamental importance were established by these classical researches.

Other important studies of metabolism were prosecuted by Pflüger and his associates in Bonn, by Zuntz in Berlin, by Tschudnovski, Pashutin, and others in St. Petersburg, by Tigerstedt in Sweden, and by many others.

The energy exchanges of the organism have a fundamental bearing in dietetics, since the heat output of the body under different conditions determines the caloric requirements of the diet. The apparatus used to investigate these exchanges, the respiration calorimeter, besides measuring the respiratory products after the manner of Pettenkofer's apparatus, determines with great accuracy the amount of heat given off by the subject. In its perfected form this mechanism is a marvel of complexity, elaborateness, and delicacy, requiring much labor and ample resources for its construction and operation.

Some imperfect calorimetric studies on animals and man were published by Russian observers from 1884. Max Rubner (1854 -) was the first to conduct a successful and elaborate series of calorimetric observations on animals. He was educated at Munich under Toit; professor at Marburg 1885-1891; at Berlin from 1891, succeeding Koch as Director of the Hygienic Institute. His studies were begun about 1889, and his results published in full in 1902. He demonstrated that the law of the conservation of energy holds good for animals; and he has laid down principles fundamental in this branch of physiology and of the utmost importance in dietetics.

The most elaborate calorimetric investigations ever carried out have been those prosecuted in this country since 1892 by Wilbur Olin Atwater (1844—1907) and his associates and successors. Atwater studied at Munich under Voit, and derived some of his ideas from Eubner. Professor of chemistry at Wesleyan University, Middletown,

Connecticut, from 1873 until his death, he devoted his whole life to investigations concerning food and nutrition. In 1892, with the assistance of the physicist Rosa, he began the construction at Wesleyan University of a respiration calorimeter large enough to accommodate a human subject. This apparatus underwent gradual improvement until finally direct determinations of the oxygen exchanges were, for the first time on a large scale, carried out. The work was jointly supported by "Wesleyan University", the Storrs (Connecticut) Agricultural Experiment Station, the United States Department of Agriculture, and (later) the Carnegie Institution. "With this apparatus an elaborate series of researches was carried out from 1892 to 1907, the results of which must stand as classical. After Atwater's death in 1907, the original apparatus was removed to "Washington and installed in the Department of Agriculture, where it is now in operation ; while his successor Francis Gano Benedict under a grant from the Carnegie Institution is continuing the research with an equipment constructed in Boston.

Other investigators have since taken up this line of work, and important points concerning metabolism under different conditions and in various morbid states are now in course of elucidation.

To recount all the important researches on the physiology and chemistry of dietetics would unduly prolong this historical review. I have mentioned the principal contributions that have first opened up the various lines of inquiry pertinent to the subject. By the researches of a host of investigators along these lines have been accumulated the data and developed the principles that underlie the theory of dietetics as we have it to-day. The evolution of the subject is still far from complete, and points of even fundamental importance are yet to be worked out. So elementary a standard, for example, as the optimum daily ration of protein, is even yet unsettled. The establishment of rational principles of feeding in disease has been very incompletely accomplished. The whole subject is in a transitional stage; investigation is, however, proceeding rapidly, and results with important practical bearings are being constantly gained.

American contributions to the subject have been noteworthy, such as the work of Beaumont, Atwater and Cannon. Honor is especially due to the United States Department of Agriculture for the special encouragement it has since 1894 given to the study of problems relating to the food and nutrition of man ; under its auspices a vast amount of research has been systematically fostered all over the country and the results published and distributed in an extensive series of bulletins.

The scientific and rational principles of dietetics have not become well assimilated into the conceptions of the public, or even of the medical profession. Dietetics is a fruitful field for fallacy, fancy and fad. There are a few diseases that have a specific dietetic treatment, such as diabetes, acidosis, scurvy, beriberi, gout, etc., in which, as also in infant feeding, the profession follows rational principles. With many diseases the appropriate dietetic principles are ignored, or have not been as yet worked out, or do not differ from those of health. In this field the dietetic management is to a certain extent a matter of caprice, guess- work and error. Faulty practises are in vogue, such as the general use as food of meat extractives and soups, although well known to be devoid of nutritive value. Mystic potencies and occult dangers are erroneously ascribed to articles of food. The distrust of food engendered in the ancient days of medicine still lingers, and there is no doubt that count- less lives have been sacrificed to the fear of feeding in disease.

The medical students and practitioners of the present and future need to be more thoroughly grounded in the scientific and rational basis of dietetics. Only by a thorough appreciation and application of its principles can this subject be raised from a position of empiricism to that scientific dignity which it is the aim of modern medicine to attain, or the powerful agency of diet be utilized in its maximum efficiency for the benefit of mankind.

Dietetic Curiosities[2]

I.

"Man is what he eats" (*Der Meusch ist was er isst*) is a German proverb, the propriety of which may be chiefly alliterative, though the apothegm of our greatest English physician goes even further: "If we could solve the problem of diet," Dr. Radcliffe tells us, "it would almost amount to the rediscovery of paradise. Wrong eating and drinking, and the breathing of vitiated air (which is gaseous food), these form the triple fountain-head of nearly all our diseases and our misery."

Even a great doctor is fallible, especially on his hobby, but it is not easy to deny the importance of a subject which can assert itself by such dire *argumenta ad hominem* as dyspepsia, congestive chills, and other penalties that follow swifter now than in old times on any violation of the physical laws of God. Love of health or fear of sickness (which differ as ancient from modern civilization) has always made the question of diet one of primary interest; yet there is certainly none about which doctors disagree more widely. It is amusing

---

[2] By Felix L. Oswald

to compare the different food-theories which have been cherished like plans of salvation since the fighting of un-nature first became a science. If contradictory tenets imply error, we surely are further from unitary truth here than anywhere except in the Babel of speculative theology; and even there only dogmatic assertion, but not inconsistency, could ever go further. Just compare the gospel of Pythagoras with that of Dr. Brown, the Berwick prophet. Abstinence from wine—alcoholic stimulants, we would say at present—and from all animal food is the keystone of the Pythagorean system, which also denounced the shedding of blood, and recommended the use of "food which needs no cooking"—fruit, nuts, honey, milk, and the like. But John H. Brown, M. D., divides all possible states of health into the "sthenic and asthenic conditions," the first to be toned down by bleeding, cathartics, etc., the second to be rallied by a liberal use of brandy and strong meats, which in more moderate quantities are to constitute our normal food, while all raw vegetable products are to be avoided, especially "acid and subacid fruit."

Is there a greater antagonism in all the *toto-cœlo* distance from Odin to Mother Ann Lee? If either was right, the other must have been portentously wrong; yet the school of Berwick, not less than that of Samos, counted its disciples by tens of thousands. Again, is there an hygienic tenet which seems more incontrovertible to us than the propriety of the three daily meals? Yet the Romans of the ante-Cæsarean era, who as physical beings were so strangely superior to us, restricted themselves to a single meal in the twenty-four hours, for which they chose the very time when we dread repletion most—the end of the day, the hour between sunset and darkness.

Moses transmits from the lips of Jehovah his by-laws against pork and rabbit-flesh, and we know how many of his followers preferred death to the obnoxious diet, but our Saxon forefathers exalted the pigs' feet of Valhalla as the supreme reward of heroic virtue, and, dying, the Baresark could grin through his tortures at the thought of celestial spareribs. Charlemagne, when informed that his life depended on a change of *régime*, declared that if he could purchase immortality by absenting himself from the customary tri-weekly barbecues, he would think the price too high. He may have doubted the efficacy of the sacrifice, but the Mingrelian ambassadors, after receiving Abu-Hassan's stern ultimatum, "Islam or the sword!" informed him that, however willing they might be to propitiate the wrath of Allah, the national assembly preferred war and pork to peace without it.

Thales considered water as the *summum bonum,* and many of his teachings seem to anticipate the hydropathic school and our temperance dogmas; but Paracelsus proclaimed to the world that he had found the true panacea and the elixir of life by the discovery of alcohol, and seems to have been only too successful in his propaganda. "He finds believers who himself believes"; and Paracelsus certainly proved personal confidence in his doctrine by swallowing (in the city of Salzburg, 1541), as the "grand quintessence of life," a five-pint bottle of alcohol, which it had taken him two months to distill. The funeral was very impressive, as the Salzburg chronicle thinks it necessary to observe. We know that our North American Indians are purely carnivorous, and persistently neglect all opportunities of enlarging their *menu;* also, that white men who voluntarily or otherwise shared their fortune and potluck for a few years, refused to rejoin Caucasia afterward. Similar stories were told in ancient Greece of the Lotophagi (lotus-eaters), a people of peculiar habits, who boasted that any stranger living among them for a little while would rather resign kinsmen and country than leave them again, only with this difference: the magnetism and the name of the Lotophagi were derived from their diet of lotus-leaves—they were strict vegetarians.

With every allowance for a possible diversity of constitutions, generic differences, and the modifying influence of climate, the subject still presents enigmas which almost force upon us the conclusion so fiercely rejected by Jean Jacques Rousseau, that nature and habit are interchangeable terms. Two hundred million Hindoos abstain from the use of animal food, by behest of Vishnu, as they say; by necessity of climate, as we explain it. But the inhabitants of Southern Africa, in defiance of Vishnu and climate, gorge themselves with meat as often as they can procure it, and with perfect impunity, it seems.

"Meat," says Professor von Liebig, "is preëminently the muscle forming food; hence the difference between the stout Briton and the lean Spaniard, the delicate Hindoo and the robust Ethiopian." But the Lesghian mountaineers and the box-carriers of Constantinople, though not vegetarians by principle, subsist chiefly on fruit and farinaceous food, and it so happens that every other man of them can shoulder a load that would task the combined strength of the stout Briton and robust Ethiopian. The powerful arms and the ponderous, leonine bearing of the occasional Turks who visit the fairs of Vienna and Buda-Pesth are a fine practical argument in favor of temperate habits; yet their rivals in strength, the iron-fisted Bauern of

Upper Austria and the Bavarian highlands, are notorious for their abject worship of beer.

But, for all that, it would be wrong to abandon the hope of rediscovering paradise by Dr. Radcliffe's road. Whatever may be the right way, we cannot afford to swerve from it, least of all consciously, and that we are astray at present is most distressingly probable. Dr. Boerhaave reminds us that there are certain maxims of health, so clearly pointed out by *a priori reasoning*, that we cannot be too cautious in the acceptance of contradictory evidence.

"For instance, the exceptional cases of robust health in conjunction with habits denounced as injurious by all analogy ought to make us inquire how this impunity is earned; which strong protector of health could overcome such an enemy. For there is such a thing as *vicarious atonement* in physiology. Athletic sports, fatiguing rides on horseback, and any long-continued exercise in open air, seem to grant a long immunity from the effects of vicious diet; and it seems that there is a peptic stimulus in mountain air and the climate of a high latitude."

The kitchen-reformers of England and North America seem united on the question of alcohol only, but contradict each other and sometimes themselves in their food-theories and general toxicology. The hygienic system of Dio Lewis embraces the vegetarian, total abstinence, and hydropathic dogmas, but in consistent logic and ingenuity is far surpassed by that of Schrodt, the Swiss dietist.

In his "Natur-Heilkunde," Schrodt distinguishes between natural, artificially adapted, and unnatural or wholly injurious articles of food. "Our natural food," he says (like Pythagoras), "are such vegetable and semi-animal products *as either are or can he eaten and relished raw, and without the preliminaries of cooking and spicing.* Such are milk, honey, eggs, nuts, cereals, a few roots, legumina, and gums, and the countless variety of fruit, which are man-food *par excellence.* Our various kinds of bread, though artificially prepared, as well as other farinaceous dishes, are derived from an edible grain which is neither repulsive nor indigestible in its original state.

"To the second or adapted edibles belong different vegetables which are rendered palatable only by the process of cooking, as cabbage, beans, peas and lentils, and various roots and leaves. Flesh, also, I will add to this list, though some would place it in the third class. Injurious, without a redeeming quality, are all narcotic and alcoholic drinks, and all ardent spices, such as pepper, mustard, and acid fluids; also those partly decayed and acid substances whose properties are more stimulating than nourishing: strong cheese, sauerkraut, and pickles."

This system is based on the idea that an unvitiated taste is a sufficient criterion of healthfulness in food, and that to the palate of a child all wholesome substances are agreeable, all injurious ones repulsive. "A taste for the so-called articles of diet embraced in my third class," says Herr Schrodt, "is always *artificially and painfully acquired.* No man of veracity or memory will tell me that he liked cheese or brandy at first." In accounting for the prevalence of stimulation and intemperance among seemingly healthy nations, he too falls back on vicarious atonement by otherwise salutary habits.

Viewed in the light of Dr. Boerhaave's theory, the gastronomic exploits of ancient and modern savages may gain an additional interest. How desirable it would be to know by which vicarious virtue his Majesty the Emperor Vitellius could atone for the often-repeated sin of devouring three brace of peacocks at a sitting, which Suetonius assures us did not prevent him from appearing in the palestra an hour afterward and joining in the games which were prolonged by torchlight toward the morning hour! Vendôme, the champion of France and the one strategic peer ever opposed to

Marlborough, was as formidable at the mess-table as on the battle-field. He would gorge himself till his joints commenced to tremble and the oppression of his chest threatened him with asphyxia. Woe to the waiter or messmate who offended him by word or want of attention in such moments! A fierce blow, a hurled tumbler, or a tremendous kick were the mildest expressions of his impatience. After the defeat of Oudenarde he saved the French army by a masterly retreat that kept him in the saddle for two days and two nights, and then restored himself, not by sleep, but by sitting down to a banquet of sixteen hours, during which he incorporated as many pounds of mutton-pie, if we may believe Chateaubriand.

Calmucks, according to Mr. Schuyler, will travel a hundred miles to stuff themselves with horseflesh at somebody else's expense; and Gordon Gumming mentions a family of Zulu-Caffres—a man, two wives, and four children—who, between noon and sunset, disposed of all the meat, marrow, and intestines of a large zebra, and during the following night picked the bones in a way which only an army of ants could emulate. Vambéry speaks of a Tartar courier, named Thuy-Kasr, who boasted of having eaten, "unassisted and without employment of witchcraft," a large skinful of raisins and a middle-sized pig, leaving nothing but bristles and a few of the larger bones; and once, within fifty hours, even a goat with two kids, together with a bag of dried figs and deep potions of *koumiss* or fermented mare's milk. Thuy-Kasr must have known the secret of Apicius, "which enabled the adept to prolong his appetite for two days and a night." But such Tartars are not the exclusive product of Central Asia. James Halpin, a Yorkshire man, who exhibited himself in Manchester and other English cities during the first years of this century, thought nothing of eating a dozen pigeons, bones, feathers and all; swallowed trout and larger fishes alive, and won a wager by devouring within two hours all the edibles, including half a cheese and a large quantity of pickles, on a table that had been set for eight persons!

Joseph Kolnicker, born 1809 in Passau, southern Germany, who served as a private soldier for a couple of years, had to be discharged before the expiration of his term on account of his appalling appetite. He would devour raw potatoes, horse-turnips, cabbages in the garden, could empty basketfuls of eggs in a few minutes, and, in spite of all precautions, gained admittance to an officer's pantry or the commissary storerooms now and then, and with most deplorable results. He, too, converted his expensive talent into a source of profit by public exhibitions, and won so many incredible bets that, much to his regret, his renown eventually spread like that of the athlete Milo, and nobody dared to challenge him.

But no modern virtuoso can emulate the giants of antiquity. Claudius, Caligula, Domitian, and Heliogabalus, the imperial gluttons, almost exhausted the resources of the Orbis Romanus by their monstrous voracity. Cicero compares the scene after a Roman banquet to a battlefield; and many of the wealthiest patricians were ruined by one or two of those entertainments, to which the above-named potentates had an unpleasant habit of inviting themselves.

The symposia of Apicius lasted from twenty to thirty hours, and his semi-annual state dinners even two days, during which host and guests were restricted to recesses of ten minutes, and etiquette required them to partake of every dish and drink, the quantity being optional, except in regard to certain spiced wines, of which a good-sized jug was *de rigueur*—a rule which could only be circumvented by liberal libations to the gods. Yet even excess itself was exceeded by the mania of Vitellius, who wasted the yearly revenue of a province on a single banquet, gorged himself for hour after hour without intermission, and, in the words of Tacitus, "unadmonished by the eruptive protests of nature, never thought of yielding while he could see and hear"! He and some of his successors on the throne of gluttony probably owed their immunity to the virtues of a long lineage of frugal ancestors. Italy, truly, is the land of contrasts, of extremes in virtue as well as in vice. The resources wasted on a single day at one of those saturnalia of intemperance would probably have fed a village for a century of the early republican era, and for at least twenty years in our present time of poverty-born frugality. Frugal, in its original sense, meant literally subsisting on fruit in distinction to carnivorous habits, which were thought extravagant. Cyrus, King of Persia, according to Xenophon, was brought up on a diet of water, bread, and cresses, till up to his fifteenth year, when honey and raisins were added; and the family names of the Fabii and Lentuli were derived from their customary and possibly exclusive diet. Eggs and apples, with a little bread, were for centuries the alpha and omega of a Roman dinner; and, in earlier times, even bread and turnips, if not turnips alone, which the patriot Cincinnatus thought sufficient for his wants. It is singular that our temperance societies direct their efforts only against the fluid part of our vicious diet; a league of temperate eaters would certainly find a large field for reform. But in Italy the thing was attempted by Luigi de Cornaro, a Venetian nobleman of the fifteenth century, who restricted himself to a daily allowance of ten ounces of solid food and six ounces of wine, and prolonged his life to one hundred and two years. Though he did not organize his followers into a sect, his example and his voluminous writings influenced the manners of his country for many years. Cornaro would not have gained many converts in Russia and Germany; but throughout southern Europe frugality, in the truest old Latin sense, is by no means rare. Lacour, a Marseilles' longshoreman, earned from ten to twenty francs a day, loaned money on interest and gave alms, but slept at night in his basket, and subsisted on fourteen onions a day, which preserved him in excellent health and humor, but got him the nickname of *quatorze oignons.*

A pound of bread with six ounces of poor cheese, and such berries as the roadside may offer, constitute the daily ration of the Turkish soldier on the march, and the followers of Don Carlos contented themselves with even less. A correspondent of the "Daily News" was served with a dish of radishes in a Catalan tavern, and ventured the remark that radishes were taken after meals in northern Europe. "You can get some more after finishing these," was the reply. The radishes constituted the dinner.

Not that men *should,* but that they *can,* live on bread alone, is abundantly proved by the records of Old-World prisons. Silvio Pellico, the Italian patriot and martyr, subsisted for seven years on coarse rye bread and water, which experience had taught him to prefer to the putrid pork-soup of his Austrian bastile. The prisoners of the Khedive were fed on rice and Indian corn, till the prayers of the French residents and his American officers induced him to sweeten their bitter lot by a weekly bottle of sakarra, or diluted molasses; and I learn from an article in a French journal that some of these unfortunates, who had passed long years without any hint of sakarra, were forced by chronic bowel complaints to return to their old dry fare.

Fedor Darapski, born 1774 in Karskod near Praga, eastern Poland, was brought to the government of Novgorod in his twenty-second year as a conscript to the Russian army, and was soon after sentenced to death for mutiny and assault with intent to kill. The Empress Catharine, acting on a recommendation of the Governor of Novgorod, commuted his sentence to imprisonment for life, but ordered that on every anniversary of the deed (an attempt to kill his colonel) the convict should receive forty lashes and be kept on half rations for a week after; the full ration being two pounds of black bread and a jug of cold water. On these terms

Darapski was boarded at the fortress of Kirilov till 1863, when at the approach of his ninetieth birthday he was again recommended to mercy and liberated by order of the present Czar.

Even the story of Nebuchadnezzar may be more than an allegory, as the wild berries, roots, and grass-seeds of the Assyrian valleys contained surely as much nourishment as sour rye-bread; and who knows but grass itself might do for a while, since the Slavonian peasants often subsist for weeks at a time on sauerkraut and cabbage-soup?

Corsican farmers live all winter on dried fruit and *polenta* (chestnut-meal), and the Moors of mediæval Spain used to provision their fortified cities with chestnuts and olive-oil. During the siege of Lucknow the native soldiers asked that the little rice left be given to their British comrades; as for themselves, they could do with the *soup,* i. e., the water in which the rice had been boiled!

But the *ne plus ultra* of abstinence combined with robust strength is furnished in the record of Shamyl, the heroic Circassian, who for the last two years of the war that ended with his capture had nothing but water for his drink and roasted beechnuts for his food, and yet month after month defied the power of the Russian Empire in his native mountains, and repeatedly cut his way through the ranks of his would-be captors with the arm of a Hercules.

The philosophers of antiquity prided themselves on their frugal habits, which ranked next to godliness in their estimation, as expressed in the famous aphorism, "God needs nothing, and he is next to Him who can do with next to nothing"—whose material needs are the smallest. Primitive habits are certainly favorable to independence, especially in a genial climate, where a man is above the fear of tyranny and all social obligations, who like Shamyl can subsist on the spontaneous gifts of his mother Earth. "Do you know," Cyrus asked the ambassador of a luxurious potentate, "how invincible men are who can live on herbs and acorns?" If the Saracens had persisted in the simplicity of their fathers, the nineteenth century might see Moorish kingdoms in southern Europe, and Arabian science and fruit-gardens in the place of deserts and monkish besottedness. Cato needed no prophetic inspiration to predict the downfall of a city where a small fish could fetch a higher price than a fattened ox.

Lycurgus, the Spartan, makes the diet of his countrymen the subject of careful legislation, but seems to have feared excesses in quality rather than in quantity: as long as the black soup and other national dishes remained orthodox in regard to the prescribed simple ingredients, free indulgence of the most exacting appetites was not only permitted but encouraged. At the philosophic reunions of the Lyceum the bill of fare permitted a choice between dried figs and honey-water in addition to the wheat-bread, which could not be refused, and Greece was the model of early Roman institutions in this as well as in other respects. Fruit and bread-cakes, spiced with Attic salt and music, entertained the friends of Plato at those suppers of the gods of three or four hours, which Aristotle preferred to so many years on the throne of Persia; but the very next generation witnessed the drunken riots of Babylon and the general introduction of Persian manners and luxuries.

The ancients undoubtedly were our superiors in hygienic insight, but among the many judicious restrictions of their dietary regimens there are some that we must attribute to prejudice or leave utterly unaccounted for. The Mosaic interdiction of rabbit-flesh, wild swan, and finless fishes has been very learnedly explained as a necessary consequence of general laws, which had to include those animals for the sake of consistency; but what on earth or below earth could induce Pythagoras, the great philosopher, to prohibit the use of *beans*—nay, even denounce any contact with the shell, the leaves, or the roots of the poor plant as a dreadful pollution? Such was the stigma he had attached to the violation of this rule, we are told, that a body of soldiers from Magna Græcia, who all belonged to the Pythagorean sect, permitted themselves to be cut to pieces or captured rather than save themselves by crossing a bean-field!

The old proverb *de gustibus* can hardly prevent astonishment at the diversity of tastes. What would Pythagoras have said about our national dish of pork and beans, or what shall we say to explain the Japanese prejudice against milk, the Papuan's partiality for fat white caterpillars, or the *gliraria* that were attached to every decent household of imperial Rome? Athenæus describes a glirarium as a large brick structure, divided by wire partitions into small cells, from five hundred to two thousand of them; every cell the receptacle of a captive rat, which was fattened on husks, rotten fish, and other offal, till a further increase in bulk would make it difficult to extract the animal through the narrow door of its cage. The perfect specimens were then collected, stuffed with crushed figs, and served in a sauce of olive-oil at the-banquets of wealthy patriots who preferred domestic delicacies to colonial imports. The Digger Indians of our Pacific slope rejoiced in the great locust-swarms of 1875 as in a gracious dispensation of the Great Spirit, and laid in a store of dried locust-powder for years to come. Even mineral substances and strong mineral poisons have their votaries. Mithridates, King of Pontus, could take a large dose of arsenic with impunity, and the mountaineers of Savoy and southern Switzerland use arsenic habitually as a safeguard against pulmonic affections. The poor Norsemen often mix their daily bread with a whitish mineral powder, more from necessity than a vitiated taste, we hope; but a similar substance is employed by the natives of Brazil and other parts of tropical America without any such excuse. The name of Panama is derived from *panamante* (originally *pan-de-monte*, mountain-bread), a substance which the Indians of Central America prepared from a mealy gypsum powder, found here and there in the Sierra. Humboldt describes a tribe of Indians in northern Brazil who have been addicted to the use of panamante for generations, and were distinguished by a monstrous protuberance and induration of the upper abdomen. When the French were masters of St. Domingo their negro slaves had contracted a similar passion, and could only be restrained by barbarous punishments from indulging it to excess.

It would be erroneous to suppose that cannibalism has become quite extinct. Among the Dyaks of Borneo there is a recurrence of the outrage after every petty feud and raid, and many of the South Sea Islands are still infested with secret anthropophagi. The Pintos, an aboriginal tribe of Yucatan, have repeatedly been detected in cannibal practices; and phenomenal cases have occurred in Asia after every protracted famine. In 1873 the Chasseurs d'Afrique captured an old Kabyle on the plateau of Sidi-Belbez (Algiers), who had committed innumerable murders to indulge this horrible passion, and had twice been caught *in flagrante* by his countrymen, who contented themselves with giving him a good hiding the first time, and released him on another occasion when they found his victim had only been a French settler!

The slaughter-houses of every large city are visited by delicate ladies, who hope to cure affections of the respiratory organs by a draught of fresh blood, but who would inspire a Hindoo with a cannibal terror more intense than that produced in the Algerian settlements by the above Kabyle. Herodotus relates that the Scythians executed their criminals by a potion of fresh ox-blood, and recommends this as a more humane method than capital punishment by the sword, though inferior to the hemlock-cup. "For opening the gates of Tartarus," says Haller, "there is nothing like a good narcotic. If I should have occasion to leave this world, I would no more think of shooting myself than of leaving town by being fired from a mortar, when I could take the stage-coach."

The Turks shudder at seeing a Frank swallow oysters, and even in the cities of Europe and North America we find individuals with similar antipathies; and I know an old professor who passed half a century in St. Petersburg, and suffered grievously from an unconquerable aversion to caviare. Caviare is the salted or pickled roe of the sturgeon—not quite so bad as Schnepfendreck, a North German delicacy, which consists chiefly of the fæces of the common woodcock.

Professor H, Letheby, food-analyst for the city of London, is responsible for the following account of a mandarin's dinner, given to an English party and some distinguished natives of Hong-Kong:

The dinner began with hot wine, made from rice, and sweet biscuits of buckwheat. Then followed the first course of custards, preserved rice, fruits, salted earthworms, smoked fish and ham, Japan leather (?) and pigeons' eggs, having the shells softened by vinegar; all of which was cold. After this came sharks' fins, birds' nests, deer-sinews, and other dishes of an appetizing and dainty character. They were succeeded by more solid foods, as rice and curry, chopped bear's paws, mutton and beef cut into small cubes and floating in gravy; pork in various forms, the flesh of puppies and cats boiled in buffalo's milk; shantung or white cabbage and sweet potatoes; fowls split open, flattened and grilled, their livers floating in hot oil, and cooked eggs of various descriptions, containing embryo birds. But the surprise of the entertainment was yet to come. On the removal of some of the flower-vases a large covered dish was placed in the center of the table, and at a signal the cover was removed. The hospitable board immediately swarmed with juvenile crabs, who made their exodus from the vessel with surprising agility, for the crablets had been thrown into vinegar before the guests sat down, and this made them sprightly in their movements; but, fast as they ran, they were quickly seized by the nearest guests, who thrust them into their mouths and crushed them without ceremony, swallowing the strange gelatinous morsel with evident gusto. After this *soy* was handed round, which is a liquor made from a Japan bean,.and is intended to revive the jaded palate. Various kinds of shell and fresh fish followed, succeeded by several thin broths. The banquet was concluded by the costly bird's-nest soup, the dessert being a variety of scorched seeds and nuts, with sundry hot wines and tea.

But the mandarin was astonished in his turn by finding ice-cream among the delicacies of an English refreshment-table, and predicted disastrous consequences from its habitual use. Ice, without doubt, is injurious, but not more unnatural than our custom of swallowing boiling-hot soups and stews.

In the use of hot spices the Spaniards and their South American kinsmen exceed every other nation. *Chilé colorado,* or red pepper, is one of the mildest condiments of a Peruvian kitchen. The *yerba blanca,* a whitish-green herb which is used raw with olive-oil on sandwiches, and enters into the composition of various ragouts, is described as resembling the *lapis infernalis* in its effect on a normal tongue. A Mexican can chew up a handful of red pepper as we would so much dried fruit, and eats onions, garlic, and salted radishes as a relief from more pungent tastes. I must believe it, on the testimony of the entire medical faculty of the city of Bremen, that a man who was treated in their city hospital for a most mysterious complaint settled the dispute of his physicians by confessing a weakness for *tan-water*—the fiery infusion of tan-bark, in which he had indulged rather to excess in the last year. The inhabitants of southern Russia, especially of the Dnieper Delta, are all day long chewing the aromatic seeds of the sunflower and different kinds of pumpkin-seeds, which appears to be less a stimulation than an idle habit, like the use of chewing gum in our boarding-schools.

Timour the Tartar celebrated his victories by solemn barbecues of broiled horseflesh and fermented mare's milk, or koumiss, which is still a favorite drink of his countrymen. Tartars also use a decoction of the poisonous fly-sponge as a stimulating beverage, and according to Vambéry have a national foible for morsels of superannuated meat, of an aroma which the French term of *haut-goût* would hardly begin to describe. Yet these same Tartars might shudder at being confronted with a dish of that Limburg delicacy which finds its way into the best hotels of Continental Europe. I cannot forget the emphatic protest of a Spanish officer who was invited to partake by a German admirer of the questionable dainty, in the cabin of a Havana steamer. "You think it unhealthy to eat that?" inquired the Hamburger, in polite astonishment. "Unhealthy?" exclaimed the Hidalgo, with a withering look and a gasp for a more adequate word—"no, sir! I think it an unnatural crime!"

II.

We know from the accounts of Sir John Ross, Captain Kane, and other Arctic explorers, how persistently the Esquimaux prefer walrus-blubber and whale-oil to the most seductive products of the vegetable kingdom, but the fervor of their devotion was only realized by the Rev. Mr. Hansen, the Moravian missionary, who prepared a dying Esquimau for the glories of the New Jerusalem. "I am sure you are right," said the departing brother, "but, tell me, are there many walruses in heaven?" "None at all, as far as I know," Mr. Hansen replied, not without astonishment at the question. The weary eyelids opened to emit a look of intense reproach. "And you couldn't tell me that before? No heaven that for me, then—an Esquimau cannot subsist without walrus!"

The peptic stimulus of a high latitude, as recognized by Dr. Boerhaave, may justify such preferences; but Greenlanders, carried down to our temperate climate and even to the eternal summers of Cuba, still insisted on their daily blubber-ration with a firmness worthy of a better cause. Ferdinand Renz, the European Barnum, found it to his advantage to gratify the national taste of his Greenlanders. He had attempted to wean them from their traditional grease, and nearly succeeded, as he flattered himself, when his managers reported an enormous deficit of tallow-candles, which he found had been devoured by the boxful in the silence of night by the bereaved children of the North.

Nowhere is indifference to the quality of food carried further than in the rural districts of Russia. Black, sour bread, salt pork, cabbage, and *quass,* or fermented cabbage-water, are the nectar and ambrosia of the Slavonic boor, who in times of scarcity will content himself with a diet that would drive Munster and Connaught to desperation. Quass, their popular tipple, is described as resembling a mixture of stale fish and soap-suds in taste, yet has next to beer probably more votaries than any other fermented stimulant.

Assassin, assassinate, and their derivatives come from *hasheesh,* the Arabian word for hemp. A decoction of hemp-leaves, filtered and boiled down, yields a greenish-black residuum of intensely bitter and nauseous taste—a stuff not very likely, one should think, to tempt a normally constituted human being. Yet this same hasheesh, Dr. Nachtigal assures us, can marshal a larger army of victims than either gunpowder or alcohol; and only the originator of the opium-habit, he thinks, will have an uglier score against him on the day of judgment than the Sheik-al-Jebel, who, tradition says, first introduced the hasheesh-habit.

The effect of this hemp-extract is compared to hydrophobia: its votaries are seized with rage and restlessness, and if the paroxysm is upon them seize a knife, a stone, or anything that will serve for a weapon, and rush out to commit indiscriminate assaults, continuing to "run amuck," as the Malays term it, till the stimulating power of the drug has spent itself, or till their career is stopped by a well-aimed shot. In Batavia and other cities of the Dutch Indies there used to be a standing reward for the slaying of a "muck-runner," but even such a man as Ibrahim Pasha was not ashamed to stimulate the courage of his soldiers by the use of the detestable poison. The hasheesh-habit originated in Asia Minor, but is now practiced throughout northern Africa down to the Abyssinian valleys, and has spread eastward to the Malay Archipelago, and even to Siam, where its further progress was arrested by the determined action of the Siamese Government.

A frugal diet has this additional advantage, that simple food is in less danger of adulteration, or must at least be imitated by equally simple and harmless substitutes. Watered milk or lard mixed with corn-meal is certainly annoying, but hardly injurious, and is a trifle altogether if compared with the abominations that are half consciously consumed by the lovers of imported delicacies and expensive stimulants. Dr. Stenhouse, of Liverpool, analyzed a suspicious sample of tea, with the following result, published in the "Planters' Price Current" of February, 1871: The package contained some pure congou-tea leaves, also siftings of pekoe and inferior kinds, weighing together twenty-seven per cent, of the whole. The remaining seventy-three per cent, were composed of the following adulterants: Iron, plumbago, chalk, china clay, sand, prussian blue, turmeric, indigo, starch, gypsum, catechu, gum, the leaves of the camellia, sarangua, *Chlorantes officinalis,* elm, oak, willow, poplar, elder, beach, hawthorn, and sloe.

There is hardly any article of food in general use which has not somewhere been converted into a stimulant by the process of fermentation. What else are whisky, rum, beer, etc., but fermented or distilled bread, the bread-corn diverted from its legitimate use to produce an artificial stimulant? Potatoes, sugar, honey, as well as grapes, plums, apples, cherries, and innumerable other fruits, have thus been turned from a blessing into a curse. The Moors of Barbary and Tripoli distill an ardent spirit from the fruit of the date-palm, the Brazilians from the marrow of the sago-tree and from pineapples, and even the poor berries that manage to ripen on the banks of the Yukon have to furnish a poison for the inhabitants of Alaska. Pulque, the national drink of Mexico, is derived from a large variety of the aloe-plant, the sap of which is collected and fermented in buckskin sloughs into a turbid yellowish liquor of most vicious taste.

Cheese, in fact, is nothing but coagulated milk in a more or less advanced state of decay. Sauerkraut is cabbage in the first stage of fermentation, which if completed yields quass, the above-mentioned Russian tonic. Chica, a whitish liquid which in Peru is handed around like coffee after meals, is prepared from maize or Indian corn, moistened and fermented by mastication.

How a fondness for such abominations is propagated can be explained by any boy who had to drink beer or eat strong cheese against his will, and by and by "rather liked it," but a question less easily answered is how such tastes ever could originate. To the first man who tasted hasheesh, alcohol, or pulque, these substances could hardly be more tempting, we should think, than coal-tar or caustic sublimate. But most articles of food and drink are older than history. All we can do is to trace their progress from nation to nation and from century to century, but their origin loses itself in the cloud-land of tradition. The exegesis of diet is as problematic as that of religious dogmas.

Natural characteristics can frequently be traced to an hereditary foible for a special diet. French wits unhesitatingly attribute the *têstes carés* of their eastern neighbors to the heavy black bread of the land of Thor, and hint strongly that the reticence and stubbornness of John Bull have more to do with his beefsteaks than with mental profundity.

"Alas, how helpless is theology against the diet of bull-beef!" writes Father De Smet in his yearly report from the Sioux missions. It certainly is a suggestive fact that agriculture had to precede Christianity in its conquests over the aboriginal North Americans. Not one of our Indian tribes would renounce the devil and all his works unless we could get them to renounce the buffalo first. I heard a vegetarian lecturer in New Orleans last year, who gave a *résumé* of the peculiar views of his people, and certainly made out a very strong case in their favor. "The aggressive, the belligerent, and bloodthirsty instincts of all nations," he said, "are exactly equal to the proportion of animal food in their diet. The Hindoos, who like pigeons seem to be 'born without gall,' are vegetarians from birth; so were the Lotophagi of antiquity, who compromised all differences by arbitration. The Malays, who, in the same climate and with the same advantages, make use of animal food, are notoriously cruel and quarrelsome. But in the Indians of North America, who are wholly carnivorous, human nature and native pity seem to have become extinct, and superseded by an artificial instinct of bloodshed which equals that of the most ferocious animals."

The Mexicans distinguish between *Indios mansos* and *Indios bravos*—tame and fierce Indians—between whom there seems to be no generic difference; but the eastern tribes are frugivorous, cowardly, and harmless as Hindoos, though in stature and facial characteristics exact copies of their western kinsmen, the flesh-eating Comanches, who in cruelty emulate the pirates of Malacca.

Erasmus complains of the porcine paunches and materialistic tendencies of his countrymen, and warns them that, when eating and drinking have become the objects of life, animalization will speedily follow.

"It was thus," he facetiously remarks, "that Circe changed the companions of Ulysses into pigs."

It is certain that the monastic gluttony of Austria, Bavaria, and the adjoining states, where plethoric convents abound, has developed an unmistakable type of grossness in the characteristic physiognomies of those countries. The *ingenium pingue* which Ulric Hutten satirizes is still an hereditary affliction in many Catholic districts, and nowhere more than in Austria proper, in Linz and Vienna, where the art of cookery has become the problem of life, and "the instinct of liberty is drowned in sausage-fat."

Abstinent habits, too, begin to set their mark if continued to the second or third generation. The ascetic vigor of Semitic countenances probably dates from the establishment of the Mosaic and Islamitic codes, with their rigid dietetic restrictions, and something in the spiritualistic eyes of the Arabian desert-dwellers suggests the absence of those animal brain-elements which according to Dio Lewis are assimilated like trichinae by the use of pork and beef. But only a French *savant* can go so far as to reconstruct the entire national history of a race from such physiognomic indications. "The face of a Turk," says M. de Chateaubriand, "shows the high cheekbones and powerful, bone-crushing jaws of the original Turkoman shepherd, improved by a diet of Attic figs and Thessalian grapes, further sweetened by the sherbet and perfumed cakes of Constantinople, and finally clouded by the fumes of opium!"

"There is a sadness in the face of the typical Chinese," writes the Rev. Mr. Gentz, "which now always moves me to infinite pity. At first they were vaguely repulsive to me, these death-head profiles and sad, sunken eyes, but I can interpret them now, and they speak to me of centuries and centuries of dull, hopeless suffering by slavery, poverty, and loathsome or insufficient food." If we believe that Dr. Fowler was able to distinguish the weavers from other operatives of a miscellaneous manufactory, merely by the formation of their heads, we cannot consistently call even Chateaubriand a visionary, for "alimentativeness" is one of the recognized organs of the craniological systems. A certain amplitude of the region between the ear and the posterior base of the skull indicates gormandism to the followers of Dr. Gall, and excessive development, therefore, of gluttony and voracity. A happy illustration if not demonstration hereof is the preserved bust of Vitellius, the imperial arch-glutton, whose enormous head seems only a reduced continuation of the still more enormous neck. Lavater, the father of Physiognomy, describes the *"Fresser-Falte"* or gormand's wrinkle which in his opinion is developed by a certain movement of the cheeks which makes us say, "His mouth waters," and by which he thinks he could detect an Austrian abbot in any disguise.

On the moral effect of sundry articles of food, Dr. Bock, the Leipsic professor, and author of the famous "Buch vom gesunden und kranken Menschen" ("Man in Health and Disease"), discourses as follows: "Flesh-food imparts courage, but also aggressive moods and bad temper, with intervals of gloom and hypochondria; excessive use of pork can produce a mental nausea, known to the Hungarians as the *Tzömör*, which may lead to insanity and suicide. The ichthyophagous tribes of northern Siberia are rendered stupid and sluggish by an exclusive diet of fish. Fish and fowl in moderate quantities and in combination with vegetable food, produce no appreciable injurious effects. The influence of ripe fruit is benign, exhilarating without the eventual reaction that always follows alcoholic excitement. Milk, too, especially the rich milk of sheep, has an assuaging, mildly cheering effect even on hypochondriacs and dyspeptics. Pure fat of any kind exercises a calming influence on excited passions, but if long continued as an article of diet tends to somnolency and lassitude. Strong cheese operates as a sedative and a check to the activity of the brain-functions—makes us stupid in other words, and can also result in a half-physical, half-psychical dejection not dissimilar to the *Tzömör*.

"Wheat-bread is neutral, a most excellent though not all-sufficient article of food, and, like a blank sheet of paper, serves as a foil to whatever you may combine it with, while sour rye-bread is a tonic and reacts on the temper in a feeble way. Eggs, raw or soft-boiled, are more nourishing than meat, stimulate muscular activity, and produce reflective rather than vindictive moods. Sugar alone, or preponderating in made dishes, causes vague uneasiness in some and merriment and wantonness in other constitutions, but moderately combined with farinaceous substances and fat, is inferior only to fruit as an alimentary corrective. Potatoes and the legumina (beans, peas, and lentils), inasmuch as they are farinaceous, are a legitimate article of food, yet not as healthy as the cereals. They lack the brain-forming elements, and, though like bread they might sustain life, they would operate depressingly—produce weariness and *ennui,* without the addition of saccharine and sub-acid food.

"The nervousness and peevishness of our times are chiefly attributable to tea and coffee; the digestive organs of confirmed coffee-drinkers are in a state of chronic derangement, which reacts on the brain, producing fretful and lachrymose moods. Fine ladies, addicted to strong coffee, have a characteristic temper which I might describe as a mania for acting the persecuted saint. Chocolate is neutral in its psychic effects, and is really the most harmless of our fashionable drinks. The snappish, petulant humor of the Chinese can with certainty be ascribed to their immoderate fondness for tea. Beer is brutalizing, wine impassions, whisky infuriates, but eventually unmans.

"Alcoholic drinks combined with a flesh and fat diet totally subjugate the moral man unless their influence be counteracted by violent exercise. But with sedentary habits they produce those unhappy flesh sponges which may be studied in metropolitan bachelor-halls, but better yet in wealthy convents. The soul that may still linger in a fat Austrian abbot

67

is functional to his body only as salt is to pork—in preventing imminent putrefaction."

Essays on diet gravitate toward the Austrian abbot, it seems. But the importance of the three daily meals was indeed wonderfully enhanced by the tedium of convent-life. The god *Venter,* Ulrich Hutten insinuates, was ever of more consequence to the holy fraternity than all the saints of the Roman calendar, and the greatest miracle in their estimation is the feeding of the five thousand with five loaves of bread. With few exceptions the abbeys and prebendaries of mediæval Europe were strongholds of gluttony, the well-appointed receptacles of the *viri amplissimi* who carved the board of the dinner-table for the reception of their ample paunches, and whose faces shone at the aspect of a favorite dish as the countenance of Moses on Sinai. Their fasts in Lent were really a satire on the *bona fide* and chronic fasts of the poor; pastry, puddings, and eel-pies in lieu of the normal venison haunches, and butter instead of ham-fat, helped to sweeten the time of penance; and Erasmus mentions the prior of an abbey who instructed his major-domo to reduce the accustomed number of dumplings for the sake of Good Friday: "Make only ten to-day," said the pious prelate—"but," after some reflection, "you can make them—a little larger."

Of what transcendent interest the bill of fare must have been to Cardinal Dubois, who called on the dying Fontenelle at his boardinghouse! The landlord announcing asparagus for dinner, and asking instructions in regard to the desired sauce, provoked an animated controversy between the two dogmatists. Fontenelle insisted on cream, the Cardinal on melted butter, till the landlord suggested a compromise—he would divide the material and use a separate sauce for each half. But Fontenelle was not destined to eat that dinner—his day of life was ended by a stroke of apoplexy before the sun had reached the meridian. Dubois, who had recognized the sad fact with a paroxysm of grief, then rushed to the landing and shouted down the memorable words, "Mettez tous au beurre!"—(Butter-sauce for the whole lot!)

Twenty per cent, of the French revenues were ingulfed by the *cuisine* of Louis le Grand, and other court kitchens have furnished very strong arguments to the opponents of royalty. During the ante Napoleonic era of small German principalities, more than one of those "commanders of four faithful square miles" astonished the world by selecting a Secretary of the Treasury from his staff of French cooks; but they who wondered did not know what secrets those functionaries could have revealed to a committee of ways and means. Peter the Great, at his departure from Castle Waldeck, where he had been feasted as the guest of the sovereign proprietor for some days, was asked to give his opinion of the château. "Everything is splendid," replied the ingenuous Russian, "only the kitchen is too large."

Such kitchens and their products have often deserved the attention of the historical pragmatist. An indigestible mushroom stew provoked King Philip's edict against his Protestant subjects and thus caused the revolt of the Netherlands, and the historical eel-pie that extinguished the house of the Medici aided the cause of the Reformation more than all the armies of Sweden and Brandenburg. Mohammed II., the conqueror of Constantinople, we learn from Raumer's history, had an attack of gastritis after finishing a highly seasoned dish of broiled liver. As a matter of course the responsible cook was put to death at once, but the pains and the rage of the Sultan were not appeased, and with his own hand he stabbed Demetrius Phranza, his beautiful favorite, son of the late chief minister of the fallen Greek Empire. By this barbarous act he alienated the hearts of his Christian subjects for ever, and planted the seeds of that hatred which perhaps at this moment bears its harvest on the battle-field of Bulgaria. That dish of sour milk and rye-bread which Charles II. had to eat in his haystack after the battle of Worcester seems never to have been digested by the house of Stuart, though it might have imparted a lesson more useful to the "merry monarch" than any precept of the Scotch Covenanters.

Frederick the Great, who proved himself the master spirit of Europe by such incontrovertible arguments, was himself mastered by his fondness for certain French-made dishes, which, according to Dr. Zimmermann, shortened his life by at least ten years. One of his odes, addressed to Monsieur Noël, his *caterer-en-chef* dwells rapturously on the merits of a peculiar partridge-pie. "Not, though, as if I doubted that such pies will send me and you *à l'enfer*" Frederick added in prose after reading this production to Noel himself. "I would follow your majesty even there," returned the courteous cook, "and it is a consoling circumstance that neither of us two is afraid of fire."

We have no Roman Pollios who chopped up a couple of young slaves every week to improve the flavor of their carps; but it is said of the Empress Elizabeth of Russia that during her residence in Moscow she caused the death of more than one courier, who had to bring in oysters and fresh sea-fish from the coast within a specified time. Domitian, the impulsive Imperator, once actually assembled the Roman Senate in special session to

71

vote on the merits of a new sauce which he desired to try on a fat specimen of *Rhombus maximus,* the Mediterranean turbot! Ælius Verus, whose administration of Asia Minor had drained the wretched province of all its available cash, spent the produce of his rapacity in less than four years in his voluptuous retreat of Daphne, or in the riots of Antioch, where it is said that a single entertainment, to which only about a dozen guests were invited, cost above six million sesterces, or nearly $240,500.

A cook in those times could of ten earn a talent ($1,200) a day, which sum, Petronius remarks, would have sufficed to hire a dozen philosophers for a year. It was the age of complete degeneration of the once so frugal Romans, who now tolerated men like Pyttilus, who got an asbestos sheath fitted to his tongue to enable him to swallow the hottest dishes and spices with impunity; or Aristolenus, who longed for the throat of a crane, that he might prolong the bliss of deglutition. Tacitus speaks of a particular dish, called the shield of Minerva, the ingredients of which cost sixty talents ($72,000), and which the ineffable Vitellius had at different times prepared at that price—an insanity which we may hesitate to believe; but less than a century ago the city of London treated George III. to a banquet of three hundred and fourteen "courses," at an expense of twenty-six thousand pounds sterling.

Opposite the Palais Royal, along the Chaussée d'Antin and on the Rue Rivoli, Paris, there are restaurants where a moderate fortune may be spent in a single week, and the *déjeuners-dinatoires* of the Frères Provençaux are not forgotten where some piquant made dishes would cost more than a year's board in the Faubourg St.-Germain.

"They offered me an *omellette* at Fitchburg," says Henry Thoreau, "an omellette with fried bacon, at forty-five cents. Not having fortyfive cents to spare for an indigestion, I bought some bread and butter, which, together with the apples I had, made me a fine dinner. We *do* need some fat and farinaceous substance once a day, but, if one can get it out of a butter sandwich and ten cents, he commits a crime against national economy and against himself if he wastes the fourfold price on an omellette and fried bacon. And why commit a further waste by calling the thing an o-mel-lette? Are not the two syllables of a pancake sufficient?"

Whatever may have been the intrinsic value of that pancake, it would certainly be worth forty-five cents to know what Henry Thoreau would have said about the following *menu* of a "little lunch," given at the Langham Hotel (London) to the members of the Dietary Reform Club (society for the introduction of horse-flesh) :

Potages—Consommé de cheval. Purée de destrier. Amontillado.
Poissons—Saumon à la sause arabe. Filets de soles à l'huile hippophagique. Vin du Rhin.
Hors d'œuvres—Terrines de foie maigre chevalines. Saucissons de cheval aux pistaches syriaques. Xèrès.
Releves—Filet de Pégase roti aux pommes de terre à la crême. Dinde aux châtaignes. Aloyau de cheval farci à la centaure et aux choux de Bruxelles. Culotte de cheval braisée aux chevaux de frise. Champagne sec.
Entrées—Petits pâtés à la moëlle-Bucéphale. Kromeskys à la gladiateur. Poulets garnis à l'hippogriffe. Langues de cheval àla troyenne. Château perayne.

SECOND SERVICE.
Rôts—Canards sauvages. Pluviers. Mayonnaises de homard à l'huile de Rossinante. Petits pois à la française, choux-fleurs au parmesan. Volney.
Entremets—Gelée de pieds de cheval au marasquin. Zéphirs sautés à l'huile chevaleresque. Gâteau vétérinaire á la Ducroix. Feuillantines aux pommes des Hespérides.-Saint-Peray.
Glaces—Crême aux truffes. Sorbets contre-préjugés. Liqueurs.
Dessert—Vins fins de Bordeaux. Madère. Café.

Buffet—Marmalade au kirsch, gâteau d'Italie au fromage de Chester, etc., etc.

The Langham has been eclipsed by some Regent Street club-rooms, if not by Delmonico's, but Paris is still the Mecca of epicures, and even during the Prussian siege Baron Brisse would have undertaken to improve on the above *menu*. Next, perhaps, comes St. Petersburg with its *mislanitza* and caviare-suppers, then London, New York, and the city that derives its name from ham-sandwiches, as Heine suggests.

The champion belt of Apicius belongs probably to Count Luckner, a Russian dignitary of vast estates in the government of Smolensk, and for a time ambassador at the court of Vienna, where he left because Herr Saphire called him an emotional swill-barrel! At his country seat of Ranzow he is said to receive a daily *programme de cuisine* from his major-domo, which he scrutinizes like the plan of a campaign. He is known to have knouted the landlord of a country tavern for using lard instead of butter in a dish of cauliflowers, and once he nearly broke the heart of his favorite cook by degrading him to the rank of dish-washer for a similar offense. "Crying and whining will not mend the matter, sir," he told the tearful penitent; "if you had assassinated your gray-haired father, I might

75

call it a perfectly natural act: but that you combine raisins and pork in the same ragout, you must ask your God to pardon you—I cannot!" At a banquet in Vienna he was able to indicate the native country of six different kinds of pheasants, but once created a sensation at his hotel by upsetting his chair and leaving the *table-d'hôte* in a towering passion— they had employed hartshorn instead of yeast in the preparation of a certain variety of sponge-cake!

Berlin has its Jockey Club and a "Hof-Restauration," and in elaborate *soupers* can dispute the prestige of St. Petersburg, but Vienna is too gross in its tastes to deserve a place in this list, though to a Hungarian palate its *gulash* (a ragout of broiled mutton) and *Kaiser-suppen* take rank with nectar and ambrosia. Quantity is prized more than quality here, as well as in other parts of southern Germany or in Bohemia, where forty men of a Prussian regiment could successively impersonate a Bohemian burgher before anything wrong was suspected. During the last occupation of Prague by the North-German troops, the legend runs, there was a grand masked ball at the opera-house, in the lower story of which a regiment of Prussian dragoons had been quartered. Somehow or other the soldiers got possession of a *domino* or complete masquerade suit, representing a fat burgomaster in his official toggery. An adventurous private donned the suit and gained admittance to the *superas auras* of the ballroom, and so on to the refreshment-hall, where his enterprise was rewarded by all the luxuries of the Bohemian season. His return to the guard-room with the tale of triumph caused a bonanza sensation, but discipline prevailed, and the regiment was organized into ten-minute reliefs, who in quick succession stormed the works and performed feats of gastronomic daring which soon drew a circle of admirers around the refreshment-table. In and out rushed the black domino, returning like Antæus with ever-renewed strength, it seemed, from a contact with mother earth. The burghers of Prague looked on, wondered, admired, and finally broke out into enthusiastic applause—they began to comprehend; it was the consistent, most natural and appropriate acting out of the part which the domino required—the character *rôle* of a fat burgomaster who alternates his official duties with short calls at a lunch-table—and only the fortieth call suggested superhuman powers and an investigation of the mystery.

North America, with all its strawberry short-cakes, clam-bakes, and railroad restaurants, is perhaps, after all, the land blessed with the most natural diet. Healthy food, which is the not-often-used privilege of the rich in Europe, abounds on the table of the poor farmer here. Our five or six largest cities emulate the vice-centers of the Old World, and have not learned yet to sin with grace and long impunity; but the populations of our glorious rural districts, in the valleys of New England, on the Western table-lands, and in the paradise of the Alleghanies, live more faithful to nature than any white men since the days of Cincinnatus, in the golden age of Italy, and in consequence are healthier and healthier-looking than any contemporary race, the peasantry of the Tyrol and the Swiss highlands alone excepted. There we meet our physical superiors; but our inferiority is not hopeless, and if we would just fry a little less and cook more, and substitute milk for coffee, Virginia and Vermont would soon turn out boys to match the prettiest Gemsenjäger of the Alpenland.

Hoeing corn and wood-chopping make a hoecake with bacon or a dish of brown beans more palatable than all the *piquanteries* of the Palais Royal; and even the hog and hominy of the poor tar-heel squatter are preferable to the Irish potato-mess or the cabbage and quass diet of Panslavonia. Exercise in open air as an aid to eupeptic beatitude ranks above all the "old reliable correctives" from the Paracelsian quintessence to Hostetter's bitters. A Persian satrap asked the Spartan ambassador for the receipt of the famous black broth of Lycurgus, but confessed himself unable to relish it without extra spices. "The spices you lack," remarked his guest, "are Spartan gymnastics and a bath in Eurotas."

In Texas, Arkansas, and the Southwestern Territories, we may find habits primitive enough to suit even a Thoreau or an admirer of the patriarchal ages. Abraham treated his angels to a *souper-dînatoire* of roast veal, barley-bread, and milk— more than the Arkansas traveler could count upon at the end of his day's journey. But the air of the prairies, Rocky Mountain adventures, or the vicissitudes of a North Carolina State road can make the homely symposion of a log-cabin as sweet as an evening with Philemon and Baucis.

It has been remarked that the yearning of homesickness is never produced by the recollection of city luxuries, but of rural diet and habits, and lonely scenery. I am often reminded of an honest mountaineer from western North Carolina who had found a position in the land-office of his State capital. After a session of the State Legislature he was standing among the spectators that always attend the arrival or departure of a Southern railway-train. "Look there, Harry!" said his companion, "there are those representatives of yours again, going to take the cars back to Marion, I guess. Don't they make you feel like taking an up-train yourself sometimes?" "Well, sir," groaned Harry, "I can stand those delegates tolerably enough, but I tell you, if I hear them cry out huckleberries in the morning, it makes me feel like jumping out of bed and starting for home, sweet home, with my shirt-tails flying!"

"Alas," sighs Montaigne, "for my own native hills, and a strawberry-patch, "*autour duquel mon âme n'a jamais cessé d'errer!*" May they flourish, the strawberries and huckleberries and the Texas pecans, the peanuts, chestnuts, and maple-trees, and the Chickasaw plums, may they be blessed! Also all johnny-cakes, corn-dodgers, and Tyrolese dumplings, and raspberry puddings, that ever restored health to a stranger or confirmed it to a native! "And above all," says Andreas Hofer in his last address to his countrymen, "beware lest they smuggle in the pottage of Esau with other luxuries of the lowlands; and let your motto be, 'Ryebread and freedom!'"

www.ingramcontent.com/pod-product-compliance
Lightning Source LLC
Chambersburg PA
CBHW050430290526
45786CB00003B/1468